Gout And

Joints

I0420739

Treating and Managing

Gouty Arthritis

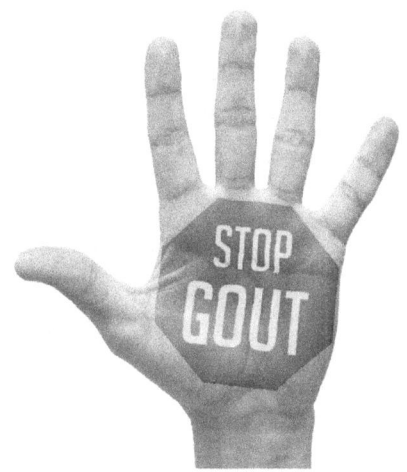

By

Paolo Jose de Luna

Paolo Jose De Luna

The information provided herein is stated to be truthful and consistent, in that any liability, in terms of inattention or otherwise, by any usage or abuse of any policies, processes, or directions contained within is the solitary and utter responsibility of the recipient reader. Under no circumstances will any legal responsibility or blame be held against the publisher for any reparation, damages, or monetary loss due to the information herein, either directly or indirectly.

Respective authors own all copyrights not held by the publisher.

The information herein is offered for informational purposes solely, and is universal as so. The

Table of Contents

INTRODUCTION 6

Chapter 1 - Gout and Gouty Arthritis 11

What Causes Gout? 16

Risk Factors of Gout 17

Chapter 2 - Signs and Symptoms 23

Having a Gout Attack 30

Seeking Medical Help 34

Chapter 3 - Diagnosing Gout and Gouty Arthritis 39

Chapter 4 - Treatment and Management of Gout 45

Treating Acute Gout Attacks 48

Managing Chronic Gout 50

Chapter 5 - Facts on Gout and Gouty Arthritis 59

CONCLUSION 66

INTRODUCTION

Joint health is one of the most important aspects of health, especially in men. As we get older, the joints grow weaker and more brittle. This occurs if you don't get adequate exercise and proper nutrition from the diet. While the joints are composed primarily of bones and bony structures, there are also ligaments and tendons that hold them together. Lacking of these connective structures, the joints would be easily dismantled and injury can result. As such, it's important that we keep these joint components healthy so that we don't suffer from ill effects from the joints such as pain, swelling, and redness.

Arthritis is one of the most common health problems that people get. With an unhealthy diet and not getting enough exercise, it's highly likely that you can get arthritis in the near future. Arthritis has three different types depending on their causes and nature – osteoarthritis, rheumatoid arthritis, and gouty arthritis.

Osteoarthritis is characterized by the degenerative process of the joints often due to aging which results in the rubbing of the bones in the joint together, causing pain and discomfort. Rheumatoid arthritis is the result from the autoimmune attack of the body, causing pain and inflammation in the joints. Gouty arthritis is caused by the excessive deposits of uric acids crystals in the joints coming from a condition known as "gout". Regardless of their causes, arthritis exhibits similar signs and symptoms which may include pain, discomfort, swelling, redness, and difficulty in moving the joint.

Gouty arthritis comes from another medical problem called gout. When an excessive amount of uric acid is in the blood, it can form into small deposit crystals that gather in the joints. Gout is commonly characterized by aching pain starting around the big toe which then proceeds to the other joints, particularly around the knees, toes, and fingers. Treating gout is essential to manage and prevent gouty arthritis and the medications for gout often correspond with those of the treatment in gouty arthritis.

As with other forms of arthritis, a healthy diet and getting adequate exercise are essential in preventing gouty arthritis. Fortunately, treating gouty arthritis isn't that hard since there are medications that can treat the condition along with different types of therapies that can help ease the pain and discomfort in gouty arthritis.

To get to know gouty arthritis, you need to know about gout first. Gout and gouty arthritis are two correlating health problems and should be discussed hand in hand to better understand the condition.

In this book, you'll be learning how to manage gouty arthritis, how gouty arthritis can begin, the signs and symptoms of gouty arthritis, how to prevent gouty arthritis from occurring, and how to manage gouty arthritis.

Chapter 1 - Gout and Gouty Arthritis

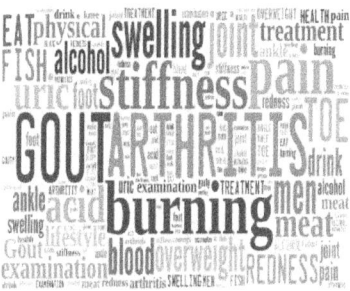

Gout and gouty arthritis are two correlating health problems. Gouty arthritis initially begins as gout which is why these two are often discussed together. The treatment options and management are also similar since they need similar medications, measures, and techniques to control the signs and symptoms. It's important to know the relationship of these two to know how to identify the signs and symptoms, as well as how to manage it properly.

Gout is characterized by a rise in the uric acid levels in the tissues and the blood coming from a problem in the body's metabolism of uric acid. Two things can bring about gout – either there is an overproduction of uric acid in the body or if there is a problem with the kidneys that result in an inadequate excretion of uric acid. As uric acid continues to build up, crystal deposits are formed and result in various health problems which include gouty arthritis, kidney stone formation, and

Gout and Joints

formation of tophi or uric acid deposits on the skin and tissues. Gout can either occur on its own as primary gout or as a result from another health problem as secondary gout.

Currently, gout continues to be on the increase when it comes to incidence, making it one of the most common health problems in the world. The complications that result from gout have also become common, making it essential to treat gout before it could even grow worse.

Gouty arthritis is form of arthritis characterized by the sudden onset of swelling and pain on the joint, most often located at the big toe of the foot. The joint may also feel hot and appear reddish, indicating the inflammatory process on the joint. As such, gouty arthritis is considered to be one of the most common forms of inflammatory arthritis that affect men over 40 years old. Gouty arthritis is often diagnosed by examining the joint for any presence of uric acid crystals through aspiration of the fluids in the joint or synovial fluid. Testing the blood to see an increase in uric acid is also helpful.

Over the years, the uric acid crystals that have deposited in the joints end up triggering episodes of intermittent inflammation.

Gout and Joints

These episodes of gouty arthritis or "flares" can be described as heating up of the joint accompanied by pain which can lead to joint damage and chronic arthritis. While gout may be a chronic and progressive condition, there are several medications and treatment modalities available to manage it even at home. Getting adequate exercise, eating a healthy diet, following the medication regimen, and following measures to prevent attacks of gout are essential in managing gouty arthritis.

Paolo Jose De Luna

What Causes Gout?

Uric acid is normally produced by the body through metabolism of the food that we eat. The tissues are processed and broken down during this phase of the cell cycle. However, those with gout either produce too much uric acid from the metabolism of the body or if the excessive uric acid is not excreted into the urine. Regardless of the two reasons, this results in the increased levels of uric acid in the blood and the tissues, resulting in a variety of signs and symptoms that indicate gouty arthritis.

Risk Factors of Gout

While gout has a specific cause and a process how it begins in the body, there are certain risk factors that may increase the development of gout in an individual. Just like other health problems, gouty arthritis have certain factors that affect their development. Here are some of the most common risk factors that increase the likelihood of gout and gouty arthritis.

- **Males** – Men are found out to have a greater risk for developing gout and gouty arthritis.

- **Heredity** – Studies have shown that if you have

parents who have gout, there is an increased chance to acquire gout as well.

- **Puberty** – Males who have passed puberty have an increased risk to develop gout compared to women.

- **Alcoholintake** – Excessive consumption of alcohol further increases the likelihood of gout because of the uric acid content in some alcoholic beverages, particularly in beer.

- **Fattydiet** – Eating too much fat in the diet can

increase the uric acid in the blood and increase the risk for developing gout and gouty arthritis.

- **Kidneyproblems**–Those with pre-existing kidney problems are at an increased risk to develop gout because they have a decreased capacity to excrete the excessive uric acid in the body.

- **Purinediet** – Eating food rich in purine like organ meats, red meats, shellfish, yeast, and certain fishes can increase the uric acid levels in the body, increasing the risk for developing gout.

Aside from the risk factors that increase the likelihood of gout from developing, there are also certain factors that can aggravate or precipitate attacks of gouty arthritis. These are often connected to the further increase of uric acid in the body and can lead to a number of complications if gout and gouty arthritis is not managed properly. Here are the following things that can precipitate or lead to an attack of gouty arthritis.

- Excessive alcohol intake
- Eating too much red meats

Gout and Joints

- Physical trauma
- Hunger
- Dehydration
- Medications
    - Diuretics
    - Anti-hypertensives
    - Aspirin
    - Allopurinol
- Chemotherapy
- IV contrast mediums or dyes

Gout is a health problem that often appears during the middle age and is more commonly identified in men compared to women. As there are several factors that can increase the development of gout, some people may actually have a normal uric acid level during their bouts of gout. Fortunately, while gout may appear to be a serious health condition, it is not contagious and can be treated with medications, as well as prevent future attacks with proper diet and exercise.

Chapter 2 - Signs and Symptoms

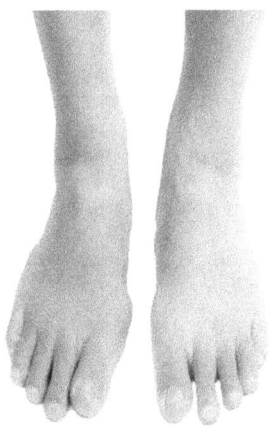

After knowing more about gout and gouty arthritis, it's time to know the signs and symptoms in order to properly identify the presence of these two health problems. As previously mentioned, gout and gouty arthritis are interconnected and it comes as no surprise that they display similar signs and symptoms.

Gouty arthritis is dependent upon the uric acid levels of the body, creating crystal deposits that can lead to the progressive damage to the joints and even the other organs if not treated in time. Here are the signs and symptoms that you need to watch out for to identify if you or any of your loved ones have gouty arthritis.

- Inflammation of the affected joint
- Stiff movement of the joints
- Joint tenderness
- Pain (often begins on the big toe)

Gout and Joints

- Kidney stone formation
- Tophi formation
- Hyperuricemia

Pain and swelling of the big toe is the most common complaint that people with gouty arthritis complain about. This type of gouty arthritis that begins in the big toe is termed as *"podagra"*. This can be accompanied with severe tenderness, discomfort, and stiffening. However, it's not just the joint of the big toe that's affected. Gouty arthritis can occur on almost any joint like the knee joint, the ankle, and even the small joints on the hands and feet. In some cases, there are those with gouty arthritis who experience pain that is so severe that even a bed sheet or the wind hitting the affected joint can elicit pain.

While the pain in gouty arthritis may become excruciating or unbearable, the first attacks can stop spontaneously without any treatment after a week or two. But even though the pain and swelling subside, the gouty arthritis often returns and affects either the same joint or another joint. That's the case when you don't seek medical treatment though.

Overtime, the attacks of gouty arthritis can increase in frequency and duration, sometimes with increasing intensity as well. The

Gout and Joints

first attacks often occur in one or two joints, however, more joints can become affected after weeks, especially without getting treatment for gout and gouty arthritis. These attacks are called *"flares"*. It's also important to remember that unseen damage can occur overtime in between flares which can lead to debilitating complications to the joints.

Kidney stone formation is also common in those with gout. That's because the presence of excessive uric acid in the body predisposes people to develop uric acid stones in the renal tract. These stones can then stay in the kidneys or block the ureters wherein urine normally passes through. Because of the blockage in the ureters and the kidneys, a myriad of signs and symptoms appear which can lead to the damage of the kidneys. If left untreated, signs and symptoms like an elevation in blood pressure, peripheral and bipedal edema, swelling around the eyes, and decreased urination can be displayed by the person.

Aside from depositing in the joints, uric acid crystals can also be found outside the joints. Uric acid crystals may form nodules in the tissues or as *"tophi"* which can often be found around the ears, hands, or elbows. Tophi are usually painful, but they are considered as an important indication of an increased uric acid level and to establish a steady diagnosis of gout and gouty arthritis. Gout can also lead to the inflammation of the fluid sacs or *"bursae"* which often grow around the elbows and the knees.

It's important to remember while the signs and symptoms of gout and gouty arthritis are largely similar, not every person may experience the same set of signs and symptoms. For example, one person may experience an unbearable pain on their joints while the other person may simply display a rise in their uric acid levels and the formation of tophi in their tissues. As such, it's essential to know when to seek medical help once you experience the signs and symptoms of gout and gouty arthritis.

Having a Gout Attack

A gout attack is often described as the swelling and pain in a joint. The pain eventually goes away, but as the gout worsens with the building up of uric acid crystals in the joints and tissues, the frequency of attacks can increase even further.

Most often, gout attacks wear off in about a week or so. These attacks can either last for several hours up to a couple of days. Without checking the uric acid levels in the blood, gout attacks may often be misinterpreted as a sprain, tendinitis, or other musculoskeletal problem in the joint. Severe cases of gout attacks can last up to weeks, leaving the joint sore and tender for as long as a month.

Most with gout experience another attack within the span of 6 months up to 2 years after their initial gout attack. However, there have been cases wherein it took many years between gout attacks. If gout is left untreated, the frequency of the attacks increases overtime and eventually the intensity of the signs and symptoms also worsen.

The first stage of gout begins when the uric acid levels in the blood rises. This may result in the appearance of signs and symptoms, but most people display no signs and symptoms at all. There are also those who have been found to have the presence of kidney stones, mostly uric acid crystals, even before the first gout attack.

The second stage of gout starts when the uric acid starts to form into crystals that deposit into the various joints in the body, often the big toe. Gout attacks begin and the affected joints feel sore, get swollen, and with varying degrees of pain. After the attack, the joint is relieved of the pain and discomfort. The gap between gout attacks may be short, but they may eventually worsen with severity, duration, and the number of joints affected with each attack.

The third stage is when the signs and symptoms of a gout attack never seem to be relieve. While some people don't get to experience the third stage because of seeking medical treatment, those who do experience it are often those who delay medical consultation. In this stage, the number of joints affected by the gout attacks increase in number and uric acid crystals may also deposit under the skin and form nodules called "tophi". If medical treatment isn't sought out, the tophi may even form on the cartilage of the ear which can cause pain, swelling, and inflammation. Overtime, gout can damage the cartilage and the bones, causing degenerative damage which can lead to progressive debilitation.

Seeking Medical Help

Knowing the seriousness of gout and gouty arthritis, one common question is asked by those who may be experiencing this health problem, "When do I go to a doctor?" Well, the answer may be more complicated than you think. While most people tend to put off going to the doctor for medical consultation because they don't experience any pain or discomfort, it's advised to seek help once you feel any form of discomfort in your joints. Once you've noticed a sudden onset of redness, swelling, or pain on your joint, seek medical help from your doctor immediately.Most often, a rheumatologist is responsible in diagnosing the presence of gout and gouty arthritis.

While the symptoms of gout and gouty arthritis may mimic those of other health problems like a sprain, an infection, or damage in the cartilage of the joints, it's important to establish a strong diagnosis of gout and gouty arthritis to ensure that proper treatment and management are given to ensure that the health of the joints are kept at the optimum level.

It's important that you should follow the medication regimen that your doctor gives you to prevent further gout attacks and prevent it from worsening. If you suspect that you may have gout or gouty arthritis, have yourself checked out by your doctor or go to the emergency room if you feel any discomfort or pain in your joints, especially when you experience gout attacks that don't respond to any kind of treatment or management measures. Further assessment and management should be done to prevent severe flares or gouty arthritis attacks in the future and promote the optimal functioning of the joints, as well as prevent the degenerative damage that gouty arthritis may cause to the joints.

There have been also reports of people experiencing abdominal pain or back pain due to the development of kidney stones from the excessive levels of uric acid which form uric acid crystals in the kidneys or ureters. If you experience any of these signs and symptoms, consult your doctor right away.

Chapter 3 - Diagnosing Gout and Gouty Arthritis

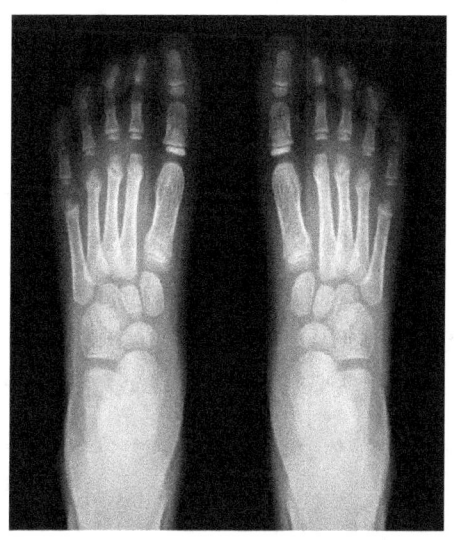

After knowing the different signs and symptoms of gout and gouty arthritis, it's time to know the specific diagnostic tests and laboratory exams to establish a strong diagnosis of gout and gouty arthritis. While it's easy to diagnose gout and gouty arthritis, it's important that the diagnosis made by your doctor has a strong foundation. That's because even though gouty arthritis may easily be displayed by signs and symptoms like pain, inflammation, and swelling of the affected joint, there are different types of arthritis that you need to be aware of which are rheumatoid arthritis and osteoarthritis.Once a stable diagnosis is established, the proper treatment options, medications, and remedies may be given to alleviate the signs and symptoms of gout and gouty arthritis. Here are some of the most important diagnostic tools to detect the presence of gout and gouty arthritis.

- **JointAspiration** – The single and most essential test to determine the presence of gouty arthritis is joint aspiration. This rules out other causes of inflammation in the joints like in cases of infection. In joint aspiration, a needle is introduced to the spaces between the joints and synovial fluid is aspirated as a fluid sample to be examined with a microscope to see the presence of any uric acid crystals, bacteria, or calcium.

- **SerumUricAcid** – This blood sample is a simple test that is done to determine the uric acid levels in the blood which is an important indicator in determining the presence of gout and gouty arthritis. This fasting blood test, though not the best indicator for gout and gouty arthritis, is still important and is quite useful in monitoring the uric acid levels to prevent future gout attacks.

- **CompleteBloodCount** –
  CBC may be done in order
  to determine the presence
  of infection to rule out
  other causes of
  inflammation in the joint
  and establish a stronger
  diagnosis for gout.

- **SerumCreatinineandBUN**
  – These two blood tests are
  prime indicators for kidney
  function which can be
  affected by gout and gouty
  arthritis with the formation
  of kidney stones.

- **X-rays** – The joint affected
  by gout and gouty arthritis
  is often visualized with an

Paolo Jose De Luna

X-ray to determine the extensiveness of the inflammation, as well as the status of the joint.

Chapter 4 - Treatment and Management of Gout

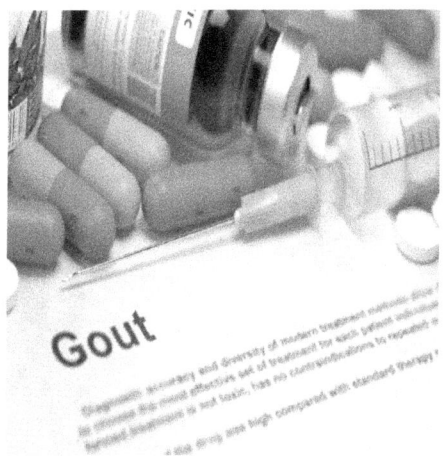

Since gout and gouty arthritis are correlating health problems, the treatment for both conditions are quite similar. Just like any other health problem, adequate exercise and proper diet still play a major role in preventing and treating gout and gouty arthritis.

Paolo Jose De Luna

After knowing the signs and symptoms of gout and how gouty arthritis can develop, it's time to know how to manage these health problems properly and how to prevent gout attacks in the future.

The main focus of treating gout and gouty arthritis is the relief of pain and prevent future attacks of gout, as well as preventing the health complications associated with gout and gouty arthritis like the degeneration of the joints, damage to the kidneys, high blood pressure, and more. Aside from exercise and diet, following the medication regimen set by your physician is important since gout is easily treated with proper medications to lower the uric acid levels in the body and utilizing measures to prevent the gout attacks that may occur in the future.

The treatment of gout can be divided into two different parts – treating the acute phase and treating the chronic phase of gout. As such, the treatment options presented here will be divided depending on the case of gout whether it is acute or chronic in duration.

Treating Acute Gout Attacks

The goal of treatment during an acute attack of gout is directed towards the relief of pain and preventing attacks in the future. At this phase, you shouldn't panic and focus on relieving the pain. Fortunately, treating an acute gout attack is easy and the measures utilized in this phase doesn't require much.

- Resting the affected joint will help relieve the pain and inflammation as movement further aggravates the signs and symptoms of gouty arthritis.

Gout and Joints

- Elevate the affected joint to reduce pain, swelling and inflammation as elevation helps in relieving the signs and symptoms of gouty arthritis.

- You can use ice to reduce the swelling since an ice compress helps in the vasoconstriction of the blood vessels in the joint and limiting blood flow, preventing the swelling from growing worse.

- Take your prescribed gout medication like NSAIDs, colchicine, or oral corticosteroids which relieve the pain and the inflammation of the affected joint. Colchicine, on the other hand, helps in eliminating the excess uric acid in the body.

Managing Chronic Gout

When gout has lasted for 6 months or more, most often when the treatment for acute gout is not followed through or if the signs and symptoms of gout persists, it is then considered as a chronic condition. Compared to having acute gout attacks, chronic gout has an increased frequency and duration of attacks or flares. At this phase, the goal of treatment of chronic gout is to reduce the frequency, intensity and duration of the signs and symptoms, as well as taking the measures to prevent gout attacks in the future.

- Take medications that are prescribed by your doctor to relieve the pain in gouty arthritis.

- Discuss with your doctor on the other medications that you are currently taking since some drugs may increase the uric acid level in the body, further aggravating gout and increasing the risk of developing more attacks in the future.

- Get adequate exercise to lose more weight and prevent future attacks.

- Limit alcohol consumption since alcoholic drinks are rich in purine which later become uric acid in the blood.

- Limit the consumption of foods that are rich in purine like red meat, organ meats, and seafood.

- Taking prescribed medications that can help

lower the uric acid levels in the blood like colchicine, xanthin oxidase inhibitors, uricosuric drugs, and other anti-gout medications.

- Resorting to surgery to remove extensive cases of tophi have developed overtime and already causes pain, swelling, and inflammation on the affected tissues.

- Drink plenty of water to help excrete the excess uric acid through urine.

- Monitor uric acid levels on a routine basis through

blood tests to ensure that the uric acid doesn't get too high as it is a key indicator in treating gout and preventing gout attacks in the future.

- Start a diet that is low in fat and in purines to reduce the increase in uric acid levels in the blood and prevent gout attacks in the future.

- Avoid fasting or diets that are very low in calories as these may actually increase the uric acid levels in the blood and may precipitate a gout attack.

Gout and Joints

- Use a cane or any support to help relieve the affected joint from bearing weight to reduce the pain, swelling, and inflammation.

- Studies have shown that cherry juice can help in preventing gout attacks as it can lower the uric acid levels in the body.

- Fresh cherries are said to have an anti-inflammatory action and can help relieve the signs and symptoms of gout and gouty arthritis.

- EPA (eicosapentaenoic acid) which can be found in

a variety of fishes, fish oils, and seaweed, is a compound that is also known to help in reducing inflammation in many health problems, including gout and gouty arthritis.

The treatment of gout and gouty arthritis relies in the person's dedication to follow through with the medication regimen and the discipline in terms of avoiding foods that can raise the uric acid levels in the body and taking management measures that can prevent future gout attacks.

Gout and Joints

If gout and gouty arthritis is not treated appropriately, it can lead to serious health complications which include joint degeneration, cartilage destruction, tissue damage, increased blood pressure, myocardial infarction, and kidney damage.

Fortunately, gout and gouty arthritis can easily be managed through proper diet, adequate exercise, and following the recommended medication regimen to lower the uric acid levels in the body, prevent the future gout attacks, reduce the pain and inflammation in the affected joints, and decrease the frequency, intensity, and duration of the signs and symptoms of gout and gouty arthritis.

Chapter 5 - Facts on Gout and Gouty Arthritis

Gout

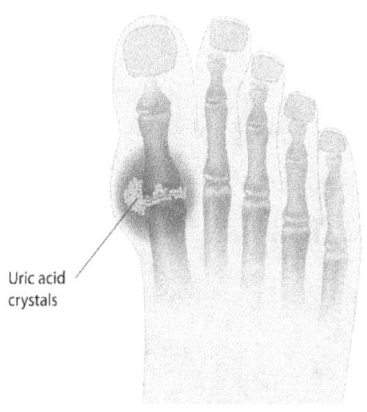

Uric acid
crystals

Because of how common gout and gouty arthritis are nowadays, there are still some misconceptions and misunderstandings about these health conditions. While they are problems that can easily be treated, some people get confused on what gout and gouty arthritis are. Here are some facts about gout and gouty arthritis that you should know.

- **Gout only affects overweight and obese people**
  - ○ Being a common misconception that most people get nowadays, gout and gouty arthritis does not only affect those who are obese or overweight as it can affect individuals

who may be of average weight or even underweight. While exercise and losing weight may help in the management of gout, the condition is highly reliant in the levels of uric acid in the blood which can rise even though you are not overweight.

- **Gouty arthritis always affects the big toe**
  - While gouty arthritis is commonly found in the joint of the big toe, it doesn't

necessarily mean that everyone with gouty arthritis experiences pain on their big toe.

- **You won't get gout if you don't drink alcoholic drinks**
  - Yes, alcohol may contribute to the increase in uric acid levels, but it won't necessarily mean that you'll be totally immune to gout if you keep off the beers and the vodka. Foods that are rich in purine like

seafood, organ meats, and red meats can increase the uric acid levels and can contribute to the development of gout.

- **Gout can't cause death**
  - Sure, it's true that gout and gouty arthritis may not really lead to death, but the problem comes from the more serious complications that develop if gout is not treated properly. This would include

complications like the development of kidney stones, hypertension, myocardial infarction, and even stroke.

- **Women don't get gout**
  - While men are found to have a greater risk of developing gout, that doesn't mean women are immune to the health problem. Gout is dependent on the uric acid levels in the body which can rise

because of the food
that you eat and the
amount of exercise
that you get.

CONCLUSION

Gout is considered to be one of the most common health problems in the world. Dependent upon the uric acid levels in the body, gout can develop into gouty arthritis which is a type of arthritis characterized by pain, swelling, and inflammation of the affected joint due to the deposits of uric acid crystals in the joints.

Gout and gouty arthritis are two correlating health problems which are easy to treat and manage. While it may bear some discomfort, gout and gouty arthritis have various ways in managing the condition which include the use of medications that help relieve the signs and symptoms of gout and gouty arthritis, lower the uric acid levels in the body, and reduce inflammation.

Just like any other health problem in the world, adequate exercise and proper diet still play a role in the management of gout and even preventing attacks in the future. It's important to have a firm dedication and discipline to follow through the medication regimen that is prescribed by your doctor and to initiate some lifestyle changes for the sake of managing gout and gouty arthritis.

Paolo Jose De Luna

If you have gout, there's no need to worry. There are a lot of ways that you can do to manage it at home and the first step that you should take is to consult your physician.

www.ingramcontent.com/pod-product-compliance
Lightning Source LLC
Chambersburg PA
CBHW071240280526
45787CB00002B/1004